WHY I HATE THE NURSING PRACTICE IN NIGERIA

Uncover the intricate challenges faced by nurses in their daily practice.

.

CYNTHIA OKAFOR ADEYERI

―――――

Edited and published by:

VITA-W Academy and publisher Abuja, FCT Nigeria.

Tel: +234 816 342 6607
Web: vitawacademy.com

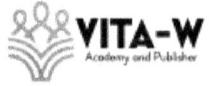

ACKNOWLEDGEMENTS

This book is dedicated to God Almighty, my family and to every healthcare professional who seeks to make an extraordinary impact on the lives of others.

TABLE OF CONTENTS

Chapter One

IN THE SHADOWS OF STRUGGLE

The Heartbeat of Care

Nursing is one of the medical professions that goes beyond medicines and procedures; it's a symphony of compassion. Nurses in Nigeria embrace their patients with empathy, from delivering newborns to supporting the elderly, these healthcare heroes play a pivotal role in nurturing the health and well-being of the Nigerian community; thereby making the healing process a journey shared. A nurse will patiently explain treatment details to a worried patient or offer solace to an anxious family member. In these moments, the true essence of nursing shines a beacon of comfort in times of vulnerability.

Regardless of these qualities, Nurses have no mind of their own in Nigeria unlike other health practitioners like doctors, they're not permitted to function without the directives of a doctor. Most nurses spend 3 to 5 years getting a formal education in nursing yet their job description isn't specified. As much as no hospital survives without a nurse, yet Nurses are not allowed to swing into formal treatment for a patient even when there's an emergency until a doctor is available. Normally Nursing has four traditional models of nursing which includes: case nursing, functional nursing, primary care nursing and team nursing.

Of these four models of nursing profession, the most prevalent in most health institutions and most preferred in Nigeria is the functional model. This method of care does not individualize care and it robs the nurse of developing skills in planning, implementing and evaluating care given to individual patients and it lacks continuity and right approach to care. This has a negative impact on best practices, standards and quality of health care rendered. The need for nurses to adopt other care approaches can't be overemphasized as it has the potential to enhance the quality of health care services.

This situation is worsened with acute staff shortage on the wards in clinics, hospitals and health care centers.

The underperformance of the Nigerian health system is caused by many factors. Among these factors are that Nigeria allocated only 5.75% of its 2023 National budget to health, which is higher than 4.76% of 2022 yet it's not up to the 15% budget as agreed upon during the African Union meeting in Abuja in 2001. This is systemic inequity in resource allocation and health workforce distribution between rural and urban health facilities, a dysfunctional primary healthcare system and a weak administrative structure of the local government which manages primary healthcare delivery. Also, the Nigerian health system is fundamentally deficient because it was inherited from the British colonial government and not planned from the bottom up to respond to Nigeria's health needs. Discriminative as it was, it catered far more to the health needs of the colonial masters and their staffers in the urban areas than to the more vulnerable rural population.

Lack of Policy

In Nigeria, nurses struggle with an array of challenges that severely affect their ability to deliver optimal health care services. One of the glaring issues is the ambiguity and inadequacy of job descriptions. Picture this: dedicated nurses striving to make a difference, yet their roles remain undefined, and burdened with responsibilities that lack clear specification. How can they excel when they are uncertain of the extent of their duties? Imagine being a nurse, eager to make a difference, but every day, your job feels like walking through a thick cloud.

Their responsibilities aren't clearly stated – it's like trying to hit a moving target while blindfolded. You want to help, but you're not entirely sure what you're supposed to do. Add to that the feeling of being lost at sea, where mistakes happen, but nobody takes responsibility for them. There's no one to say, "This is where things went wrong, let's fix it." It's like trying to navigate a puzzle in the dark without any hints or signs. The absence of upholding a culture of accountability further the turmoil within the nursing profession. Nurses are left adrift in the sense that they could barely tell what their exact job is. The lack of clear structures for better understanding of their responsibility can lead to situations where mistakes could barely be traced to its origin, thereby inhibiting growth, improvement, and learning.

Identity crisis looms over nurses like a shadow, casting doubt upon their purpose and their place within the healthcare ecosystem. They're left with a profound struggle to find their niche, to understand where they belong in the complex web of healthcare delivery. This identity crisis robs them of confidence and direction, leaving them to wander in a wilderness of uncertainty. And it's not just about not knowing your role – it's also feeling like you don't really know who you are in the healthcare system. You're a nurse, yes, but where do you fit? What's your place in the grand scheme of things? That uncertainty creates a feeling of being lost, unsure of which path to take.

Amidst this turmoil, nurses find themselves unsure of what actions to take or how best to serve their patients. The absence of clear guidance and support leaves them stranded, hence they struggle with the ethical quandaries without a compass to guide their decisions. Nurses are faced with tough decisions every day, but they are not sure if what they're doing is the best thing for their patient. It's sad that in Nigeria, there's no Nurse clear guidebook, no set of instructions to follow. It's like trying to solve a puzzle without knowing what the picture is supposed to look like, who can do that? The stifling lack of autonomy within the nursing profession shackles these caregivers. Nurses, who possess a wealth of knowledge and expertise, are bound by restrictive

7

protocols and bureaucratic red tape. There's this sense of having a toolbox full of tools, but being told you can only use a few tools, same goes to the nursing profession, they're equipped with the skills and knowledge yet their practice is limited. As a Nurse, you want to use your skills, your judgment, to make a real difference to cater to your patients' needs with discretion and wisdom, only to realize you are constrained, your hands are tied, you can't fully practice in the best interest of those you serve. There are rules and protocols holding you back from providing systemic and tailored care.

This restriction doesn't just affect nurses; it affects the care patients receive. Imagine if you could give more, if you could provide care tailored to each person's needs. It's not just about doing a job; it's about making sure people get the best care possible when they need it the most. It's a disheartening plight that hampers the very essence of compassionate caregiving and stunts the growth of a profession that should flourish. In the healthcare hierarchy, nurses are often relegated to a position where their voices are stifled, and their contributions are overshadowed by other health care service providers. Their potential to offer valuable insights and make critical decisions for the well-being of their patients is curtailed. Instead, they find themselves bound by the rigid constraints of following directives issued by doctors, leaving them feeling voiceless and without autonomy.

This lack of autonomy not only diminishes the value of the nursing profession but it also deprives patients of the comprehensive care they deserve. Imagine a scenario where nurses, equipped with vast knowledge and compassionate hearts, yet they'll stand bedside, yearning to offer personalized care to their patients. In this landscape, doctors reign supreme, holding the key to every patient's fate.

9

Nurses, despite their expertise, are relegated to mere executors of orders, trapped in a cycle that undermines their professional worth.

The prevailing sentiment among nurses echoes a weaponized truth: a feeling of being caged within the confines of doctor-led directives. We yearn to contribute more, to offer care that transcends the routine administration of injections. Our longing is not merely for recognition but for the ability to make meaningful contributions to our patients' well-being. The perception that nursing is merely about administering injections or carrying out orders undermines the extensive knowledge, skills, and dedication that nurses bring to their profession. They are so much more than that - Nurses are compassionate caregivers, advocates for patient well-being, and knowledgeable professionals capable of making significant contributions to healthcare.

Of truth, nurses are driven by a passion for healing and caring, however they find themselves constrained by a system that fails to recognize their expertise and potential. The adage "you can't give what you don't have" rings true here – without the freedom to exercise their skills and judgment, nurses are unable to offer the level of care that aligns with their training and dedication. What does it mean to be a nurse in such an environment? It means struggling to find one's identity amidst the shadows of hierarchical dominance. It means yearning to provide individualized care, yet being bound by a system that values conformity over innovation. Nurses find themselves caught between their aspirations to excel and the harsh reality of limited autonomy.

The plight of nurses in Nigeria embodies a larger narrative, one of it is where the healing touch of compassionate caregivers is restrained, where their potential to transform lives is hindered by systemic constraints. Their struggle is not merely for personal recognition; it's a plea for a healthcare system that values their expertise and empowers them to be the change-makers they aspire to be.

Nurses have to get their own goals and objectives straight;

- Who are you as a nursing professional?

- What do you do?

- What does society stand to gain from you?

When I mention my profile to people, they think I have been able to attain all my milestones because I am rich, or because I am connected to people at the top, but it is not so. Being a Registered nurse who is skilled, with a solid track record in Acute Care, Med Surgery, Pediatrics, Accidents and Emergencies, and Nursing Management. I graduated from the State School of Nursing in Delta State and I went on to obtain Leadership Certifications from the University of Washington, Great Learning and Alison.

Currently I am driving the UN's 2030 agenda through SDGs 1, 3, 4, as stated earlier, I didn't get here by merely wishing only; before venturing into nursing, I clearly set what goals I plan to achieve as a Nurse. I started by working towards changing the narrative. I didn't want to follow the status quo because I didn't choose nursing asthmatics or title, I truly want to make a healthy living a lifestyle.

I made it clear to myself that I want to make a difference, this is what a lot of nurses lack. The charge to drive change and make positive differences, not just to do a job. A lot will change in our work setting when we adopt this principle. We will stand out when we take this initiative.

Nursing professional in Nigeria is more than a caretaker or a follower of directives. Nurses are beacon of hope, guardian of health, and a catalyst for change. They embody compassion, expertise, and an unwavering commitment to the well-being of every individual who crosses their path. They're not merely nurses; they're advocates for holistic care, relentless seekers of knowledge, and staunch supporters of patient empowerment. Nurses are the soothing voice in times of distress, the reassuring presence in moments of uncertainty, and the guiding hand navigating the complexities of healthcare.

As far as Professional Nursing is concerned, you'll agree with me that the role transcends the routine administration of medications or the execution of doctor's orders. They're healers with a profound understanding of the human condition, mind, body, and soul. Nurses listen intently, assess meticulously, and act decisively to alleviate pain, promote wellness, and restore dignity. Society stands to gain immensely from the nursing professionals, because they bridge the gap between healthcare systems and the community, they facilitate health literacy, promote preventive care, and are a champion of overall well-being. Nurses also double as educators; they empower individuals to take charge of their health by guiding them towards healthier lifestyles and disease prevention. The contribution of nursing professionals extends beyond the walls of hospitals and clinics, they advocate for health equity, crusade against systemic injustices.

Nurses bring positive change to health, wellness, and equality of the citizens in diverse societies. Therefore, Nurses shouldn't be merely defined by the limitations imposed upon me.

Just like every other nurse out there, my aspirations goes beyond personal recognition; they are rooted in a fervent desire to be an agent of change, to revolutionize healthcare systems, and to elevate the standards of care for every individual in Nigeria. In essence, Nurses are steadfast advocates for compassionate care, a relentless pursuer of excellence, and a beacon of hope for a healthier, more equitable future.

Chapter Two

A SYSTEM IN CRISIS

I n the realm of healthcare, the stark contrast between practices in the Western world and the Nigerian healthcare system speaks volumes about the difference in standards and structural organization. Hospitals in the Western world, are regarded as citadel of care, they prioritize patient safety by restricting visitor access to the wards. This measure isn't merely about protocol; it's a strategic process aimed at curbing infections and safeguarding both patients and visitors from potential health hazards.

In Western hospitals, visitors are redirected away from the wards, maintaining a strict boundary between patients and potential contaminants. This thoughtful approach prevents the transmission of infections like the dreaded nosocomial infections, commonly known as hospital-acquired infections. Hospitals are equipped with comprehensive facilities and resources, ensuring patients receive necessary care without external exposure to contagious elements. This practice, rooted in infection control protocols, emphasizes the critical need to maintain a sterile environment for patient recovery.

However, the Nigerian healthcare system stands in stark contrast. Here, the lack of structured protocols creates an environment where visitors freely wander through hospital wards, often oblivious to the risks they pose to both patients and themselves. This absence of strict visitor regulations is a typical issue.

A healthcare infrastructure struggling to meet international standards. The absence of training programs for nurses on effective communication with patients' relatives and friends worsens the situation. In this vacuum of guidance and structure, interactions often lack professionalism, leading to instances where nurses might inadvertently come across as rude or mannerless.

A concerned friend or relative arrives at a hospital in Nigeria, seeking solace in visiting their ailing loved one. However, they are greeted not by empathetic and informative guidance from healthcare providers but by a disorganized environment and a lack of clear communication. Without proper guidance, visitors inadvertently become potential carriers of infections, posing risks to patients and themselves. In Nigeria's healthcare landscape, the absence of standardized visitor management practices underscores the pressing need for reform. The absence of robust training programs for nurses not only diminishes professionalism but also endangers the well-being of patients and visitors alike.

This scenario sheds light on the obvious reality: an empty vessel cannot pour forth knowledge. In the absence of structured systems and standardized practices, the vacuum created is filled with uncertainties, risks, and missed opportunities for improvement. The root cause lies not only in the demeanor of nurses but in the systemic deficiencies that fail to provide adequate training and support. It is imperative to equip nurses with the tools, training, and protocols necessary to navigate complex interactions with patients' relatives in a manner that is both compassionate and effective. Only through structured education and guidance can nurses effectively manage these situations, fostering an environment conducive to patient recovery while ensuring the safety of all involved.

The healthcare system in Nigeria cries out for structured protocols, comprehensive training, and a paradigm shift towards patient safety and professionalism. Only then can we bridge the gap between the chaos of the present and the standards of global healthcare excellence.

Knowledge is the cornerstone of professional competence, yet it's the fusion of expertise with empathy that elevates healthcare services to an exceptional standard. Beyond technical expertise, the ability to connect with patients and their families on a personal level, elevates the quality of service provided by healthcare professionals. The significance of empathy, compassion, and effective communication cannot be overstated. In the realm of patient care, a warm, jovial demeanor can be as potent as any medication. The ability to interact with patients and their families in a compassionate, empathetic manner not only fosters trust but also significantly impacts the overall experience of healthcare delivery.

Consider the scenario of delivering a life-altering diagnosis, such as informing an individual about their HIV status. The manner in which this delicate information is conveyed holds immense significance. Approaching this conversation with empathy, sensitivity, and a supportive attitude can make a profound difference in the patient's acceptance, understanding, and subsequent adherence to treatment.

The physical environment of healthcare facilities plays a pivotal role in the healing process. Hospitals are more than just spaces for medical treatment; they are sanctuaries for healing and recovery. The incorporation of well-designed sections like cafeterias, libraries, and lounges within hospitals transforms the ambiance, offering patients and their families areas for respite and relaxation. Imagine strolling through a hospital's lush garden filled with therapeutic plants and flowers. The serene sight, coupled with the calming fragrance and natural elements, creates an environment conducive to healing. Trees, flowers, and greenery have been proven to have therapeutic effects, reducing stress, promoting healing, and contributing to an overall sense of well-being. These initiatives go beyond aesthetics; they foster an atmosphere conducive to healing and recovery.

While these might seem like luxuries, they are indeed whole components of healthcare that should be embraced and implemented, even in Nigeria. Hospitals should not be merely clinical spaces but sanctuaries that promote healing on multiple levels; physically, emotionally, and psychologically. In Nigeria, the transformation of healthcare facilities to incorporate these elements might initially seem impossible, however, it is entirely feasible. By recognizing the importance of a conducive environment for healing, hospitals can strategize and invest in creating therapeutic environments. Initiatives to plant therapeutic gardens, establish comfortable lounge areas, and integrate spaces that foster relaxation and distraction can significantly enhance the overall patient experience.

Ultimately, investing in these elements isn't just about aesthetics; it's about recognizing the profound impact they have on the well-being of patients, their families, and even healthcare providers. It's a step towards creating an environment that nurtures healing, promotes recovery, and uplifts spirits, a space where both physical and emotional health converge for a better approach to healthcare. It's time for Nigerian hospitals to embrace these innovative approaches, creating spaces that promote healing, comfort, and rejuvenation, ultimately fostering an environment where healthcare isn't just about treatment but about whole care for the mind, body, and spirit.

Chapter Three

BEYOND THE BEDSIDE: THE UNSEEN BURDEN

The unseen burden in the health care goes beyond the bedside conduciveness. The commitment made by the Nigerian government to allocate 15% of its annual budget to the health sector, as agreed upon during the African Union meeting in Abuja in 2001, stands as a reminder of an unfulfilled promise. Fast forward to the present, and the reality contrasts with this pledge. Despite the gap of 22 years since this commitment, the desired allocation to healthcare remains a distant dream. The underfunding of the healthcare system in Nigeria poses a significant challenge. The promised 15% allocation, if realized, would have had transformative effects, ensuring improved infrastructure, access to essential medications, advanced medical equipment, and a well-equipped workforce. However, the persistent shortfall in budgetary allocations hampers progress and perpetuates deficiencies within the healthcare sector.

Statistics paint a distressing picture. Despite the recognized need for substantial investment in healthcare, Nigeria's allocation to the sector has consistently fallen far below the pledged 15%. Consider this: Nigeria allocated only 5.75% of its National budget to health, which although higher than 4.76% of 2022 remains alarmingly low compared to global standards. For a nation with a population that exceeds 200 million people, the inadequate budget allocation to healthcare raises concerns about the ability to meet the diverse health needs of its populace. According to data, Nigeria's healthcare expenditure accounted for only a fraction of its GDP, lagging significantly behind the recommended levels by global health organizations.

The consequence of this underfunding situation throughout the healthcare system. Hospitals and clinics struggle with insufficient resources, leading to shortages of essential medications, medical equipment, and adequately trained healthcare professionals. The burden falls on the shoulders of both patients and healthcare workers, grappling with the ramifications of a system in dire need of support. Many Nigerians, particularly those in rural areas and underdeveloped communities, face insurmountable barriers to accessing healthcare due to the extravagant cost of services. A subsidized healthcare system would alleviate the financial burden on individuals and families, ensuring equitable access to essential medical care for all.

Subsidizing the cost of healthcare services becomes paramount in a scenario where budgetary allocations fall short. The implementation of subsidies could alleviate the financial strain on individuals seeking medical care, ensuring that quality healthcare remains accessible and affordable for all segments of society, particularly the vulnerable and marginalized.

To address these systemic challenges, the government must take proactive steps. Establishing a dedicated regulatory body tasked with overseeing healthcare operations and ensuring accountability becomes imperative. This body, operating with transparency, will conduct regular assessments, and implement policies that prioritize the well-being of citizens. Such an entity would be responsible for ensuring the effective utilization of resources, thereby maintaining quality standards, and implementing strategic initiatives aimed at improving healthcare delivery nationwide.

It would serve as a beacon of accountability, ensuring that allocated funds are utilized efficiently and transparently for the benefit of the population.

Furthermore, sufficient budgetary provisions are crucial for the effective functioning of the healthcare system. Increased funding can aid infrastructure development, enhance medical facilities, and facilitate comprehensive healthcare delivery. Investment in healthcare is an investment in the nation's future, a healthy populace drives economic growth, social stability, and national prosperity. It's time for Nigeria to uphold its commitment to allocate 15% of its annual budget to healthcare. This pledge, if fulfilled, holds the potential to transform the healthcare landscape, ensuring that every citizen has access to quality, affordable healthcare which is a fundamental right that should not be compromised.

The departure of pharmaceutical giant GSK from Nigeria is indeed a wake-up call, urging us to seize the opportunity to cultivate a self-sufficient healthcare system. In the absence of major international players, the onus falls on Nigeria to foster a robust system for generating and manufacturing drugs and medicines domestically. Embracing local production of drugs and medicines is not merely a necessity but a strategic imperative for ensuring healthcare resilience and sustainability.

The vast reservoir of traditional medicine in Nigeria offers a promising avenue to tap into. Traditional medicine, deeply rooted in our culture and heritage,

31

holds untapped potential. Integrating traditional healing practices with modern pharmaceutical techniques can unlock the treasure of remedies, offering solutions to various health challenges. Exploring and harnessing traditional medicinal knowledge requires a concerted effort to bridge the gap between ancient wisdom and modern science. Collaborative research initiatives can help validate the efficacy of traditional remedies, identifying active compounds and formulations that could serve as the basis for developing new drugs.

By leveraging scientific research and technological advancements, traditional medicine can be studied, refined, and standardized to create effective, evidence-based pharmaceuticals.

Nigeria boasts a rich biodiversity, with an abundance of medicinal plants and herbs used for centuries by indigenous communities. These natural resources harbor compounds with therapeutic properties that, if properly studied and refined, could lead to the development of novel drugs and treatments. Imagine the possibilities of integrating indigenous knowledge with modern pharmaceutical technologies to refine and enhance the efficacy of traditional remedies. Investing in machineries and technologies for refining locally sourced medicinal compounds can play a pivotal role in making these remedies more appealing and marketable. By employing modern refining processes, we can elevate the quality, purity, and standardization of traditional medicines, thereby making them more acceptable in both local and global markets.

However, to achieve this transformation, concerted efforts are required. Collaboration between government bodies, research institutions, pharmaceutical companies, and traditional healers is crucial. Establishing research centers or institutions dedicated to the study of traditional medicine could serve as hubs for scientific exploration and development. This will go a long way along with setting up initiatives to train and empower local researchers, could pave the way for innovation and progress in this domain.

These centers could delve into the chemical compositions of traditional remedies, identify active ingredients, and conduct clinical trials to validate their desired effect. Additionally, regulatory frameworks should be put in place to ensure quality control, standardization, and safety of locally produced medicines. This instills confidence among consumers and facilitates market penetration for these products.

The refinement of locally sourced medicinal ingredients is pivotal in enhancing their appeal and marketability. Investing in machineries and technologies for refining, processing, and standardizing these raw materials can elevate their quality to meet global standards. By adopting sophisticated refining processes, indigenous medicinal products can compete on par with Western drugs, thus increasing their desirability. You should note that this shift towards local pharmaceutical production isn't solely about economic viability; it's also about fostering self-sufficiency and promoting the health and well-being of the population. The reliance on imported drugs not only strains the economy but also leaves the nation vulnerable to supply chain disruptions and price fluctuations.

For instance, the global COVID-19 pandemic exposed the vulnerability of nations reliant on imported drugs, emphasizing the urgent need for self-reliance in pharmaceutical production. Nigeria's quest to develop its pharmaceutical industry aligns with global trends towards self-sufficiency and resilience in healthcare. Nurses should be encouraged to go into research and see how to contribute to the pharmaceutical field, not just doctors and pharmacists. Nurses can also work in that line, to identify effects and results of medications on children. We work towards the betterment of our system, and how to modify what we do here. In essence, the departure of GSK serves as a clarion call for Nigeria to chart its path towards pharmaceutical self-sufficiency. By tapping into our rich tradition of healing practices, investing in research, and leveraging modern technologies, we can revolutionize the healthcare landscape, offering innovative, effective, and locally produced drugs that cater to the needs of our people and beyond.

Chapter Four

THE TRAINING GROUND: AN UPHILL BATTLE

The Nursing Council of Nigeria was established in 1949 to coordinate the schools of nursing and create standards for nursing education and practice. The programmes offered by the schools were either basic or post basic in nature. The programme includes; general nursing (3 years/18 months); midwifery (3 years/1 year); psychiatry nursing (3 years/1 year) respectively either as basic or post basic. The academic curricula were reviewed severally in response to the needs of the society. Certificates offered by the three year nursing diploma programmes have recently been quantified for promotion purposes and judged to be equivalent to a Higher National Diploma Certificate to fall in line with the education and civil service structures in Nigeria.

There are a variety of nursing career paths in the healthcare field. The requirements for education and training vary for each role, as well as the responsibilities and skills needed in that position. Here are some nursing common career professions obtainable in Nigeria:

- Certified Nursing Assistant (CNA)

- Licensed Practical Nurse (LPN)

- Registered Nurse (RN)

- Certified Registered Nurse Anesthetist (CRNA)

- Clinical Nurse Specialist (CNS)

- Nurse Practitioner (NP)

The most common specialty is the Registered Nurses, there are over 180,000 RNs in Nigeria, to cater to a population of over 200 million. Do the math and calculate the ratio, see what you will get. But that's not even the point. The common steps you can take to become an RN include:

- Complete an accredited nursing education program—RNs may either earn an associate degree in nursing or a Bachelor of Science in nursing from an accredited nursing school.

- Pass the National Council Licensure Examination for registered nurses.

- Become licensed.

To move up the ladder, you must jump some more serious hurdles specific to the career path you chose. It is never easy. In these times and age, the commodification of nursing education into short, condensed programs, often claiming to transform individuals into certified nurses within a mere three months, is a disheartening trend that compromises the integrity of the nursing profession. This shortcut approach undermines the essence of nursing, which demands comprehensive education, practical training, and a deep understanding of medical and ethical complexities. In Nigeria, and indeed in many parts of the world, there exists a misconception that nursing can be mastered within an incredibly short period. Some individuals or institutions capitalize on this misconception, offering quick, crash-course programs that promise to churn out certified nurses within a fraction of the time required for a proper nursing education.

Consider the gravity of this situation: nursing is a profession that demands not only technical skills, such as administering injections or inserting cannulas, but also requires a profound understanding of anatomy, physiology, pharmacology, psychology, and ethics, among other disciplines. Nursing education encompasses a wide array of theoretical knowledge, clinical skills, critical thinking, and ethical understanding.

The foundational principles of nursing—holistic care, patient advocacy, evidence-based practice, and comprehensive assessment, cannot be condensed into a mere three-month crash course. Nursing education traditionally involves rigorous academic coursework, practical clinical experiences, and a period of supervised training to develop competent and compassionate nurses.

In this rush for quick certifications, the focus often narrows down to basic procedural skills like inserting a cannula, administering injections, or setting up IV drips. While these skills are integral parts of nursing practice, they represent only a fraction of the multifaceted responsibilities that a qualified nurse must handle. Nursing is not just about performing tasks; it's about understanding the underlying pathophysiology, patient assessment, critical decision-making, and providing well-tailored care to individual needs. The misrepresentation of nursing as a skill that can be acquired in a few short months undermines the essence of the profession.

It belittles the dedication and commitment required to become a proficient nurse, devaluing the significance of a patient's care and critical thinking skills.

These abbreviated programs often lack accreditation or regulatory oversight, leading to a scenario where individuals may possess rudimentary technical skills but lack the essential knowledge, critical thinking ability, and ethical foundation that define a well-rounded nurse. Such a scenario poses serious risks to patient safety and quality of care. Moreover, these quick-fix certification courses devalue the years of dedication, hard work, and rigorous education that certified nurses undergo. Nursing is a noble profession that demands in-depth knowledge, continuous learning, and a commitment to ongoing professional development.

Diluting the essence of nursing education by condensing it into a short duration diminishes the credibility of the profession and erodes public trust in the healthcare system. The issue extends beyond the immediate consequences for patient care. It impacts the entire healthcare ecosystem, contributing to a culture where shortcuts overshadow competence, leading to a decline in healthcare standards and professionalism. In the pursuit of quick monetary gains, these abbreviated nursing programs perpetuate a cycle of unprepared, underqualified individuals entering the healthcare workforce, ultimately compromising the credibility and standards of the nursing profession.

To maintain the integrity of nursing and uphold the quality of patient care, it is imperative to emphasize the importance of comprehensive, accredited nursing education that adheres to established standards and regulations. To safeguard the integrity of the nursing profession, regulatory bodies, educational institutions, and policymakers must step up. They need to enforce stringent accreditation standards for nursing education programs, cripple all illegal institute and hospitals, emphasizing comprehensive curricula, clinical experiences, and assessments that truly prepare individuals for the multifaceted responsibilities of nursing. Professional bodies should advocate for the recognition and respect of the nursing profession, highlighting the depth of knowledge and skills required to deliver quality care.

Additionally, public awareness campaigns can help dispel misconceptions about the complexities of nursing and educate the populace about the importance of seeking care from qualified healthcare professionals.

Raising awareness about the essential components of a proper nursing education, advocating for the value of comprehensive training, and fostering a culture that values expertise over shortcuts are critical steps in safeguarding the integrity of the nursing profession and, most importantly, ensuring the safety and well-being of patients.

Chapter Five

THE TOLL OF MENTAL HEALTH

The repercussions of the flawed nursing education system in Nigeria resonate far beyond inadequate training, it manifests as a heartbreaking tale of qualified nurses relegated to the sidelines, their expertise overlooked and their aspirations unfulfilled. The dire state of affairs within the healthcare system leads to the disenfranchisement of these skilled professionals, leaving them grappling with feelings of depression, disillusionment, and a sense of being undervalued.

Qualified nurses, who are experienced with knowledge, skills, and a fervent passion to make a difference in patient care, find themselves constrained within a broken system. They face significant barriers that prevent them from practicing their specializations or utilizing the depth of their expertise. Instead of being recognized and appreciated for their gifts, they encounter a landscape where their potential remains largely untapped and underutilized.

Some Nurses have invested years of dedication, financial resources, and untold sacrifices into acquiring their qualifications. Their dreams of making meaningful contributions to healthcare are stifled within a system plagued by inefficiencies, lack of recognition, and disregard for professional speciali-zation. The result? A workforce of highly skilled and motivated individuals, who, due to systemic limitations, seek opportunities abroad not solely for greener pastures but for the chance to apply their ex-pertise in environments that acknowledge and value their contributions. It's not a flight from homeland but rather a quest for professional fulfillment and recognition.

The journey to become a nurse is one of the demand-ing academic study, practical training, millions of Naira and personal sacrifice. Yet, the unfortunate re-ality is that many of these dedicated professionals find themselves trapped in a system that fails to pro-vide them with avenues to leverage their expertise effectively. Moreover, the increasing levels of pov-erty in Nigeria add a layer of complexity to this pre-dicament. Nurses, driven by their passion for their profession, struggle amidst economic hardships, often facing financial constraints that compound the challenges they encounter within the healthcare system. The systemic deficiencies not only impact individual nurses but also have far-reaching implications for patient care and the healthcare system at large. The potential of highly qualified nurses remains largely untapped, depriving patients of the full spectrum of care they could receive if these professionals were allowed to practice to their fullest potential.

The plight of nurses in Nigeria extends beyond professional limitations; it's a struggle for survival, dignity, and the ability to utilize their hard-earned skills. The financial hardships faced by nurses is one of the challenging situations, which has made many unable to adequately support themselves and their families. These financial constraints create a barrier that prevents them from pursuing further studies or seeking opportunities abroad to advance their careers.

The accumulation of these challenges compounds the distress experienced by nurses, leaving them in a state of perpetual frustration and despondency. Their noble aspirations to serve the community through nursing are thwarted by a system that doesn't appreciate or acknowledge their expertise. Instead of fulfilling their roles as skilled healthcare providers, many find themselves relegated to menial tasks like sweeping hospitals and undertaking cleaning duties that don't align with their training or qualifications. Imagine the emotional toll this could take on nurses?

Their dreams of making a meaningful difference in people's lives through healthcare provision are hindered, and their professional aspirations are thwarted by the limitations imposed upon them. The inability to practice what they have studied for years not only affects their self-worth but also impacts their mental and emotional well-being.

The sense of underappreciation affects every aspect of their professional lives. Nurses, armed with extensive knowledge and skills acquired through rigorous education, find themselves constrained, unable to exercise their professional judgment or contribute meaningfully to patient care. The frustration of being unable to utilize their position and power as nurses leaves them feeling handicapped, demotivated, and constantly questioning their career choices. This situation is not just disheartening for individual nurses; it's detrimental to the healthcare system as a whole. A workforce of highly qualified, skilled nurses constrained from practicing to their full potential hampers the delivery of quality healthcare services, affecting patient outcomes and eroding trust in the healthcare system.

The emotional burden of being undervalued, the mental strain of being unable to fulfill their professional potential, and the financial struggles to make ends meet paint a grim picture of the reality faced by many nurses in Nigeria. The ripple effect of these challenges permeates through the fabric of society, impacting families and communities. Addressing these issues requires a systemic overhaul, one that recognizes and values the expertise of nurses, provides opportunities for their professional growth and development, ensures fair compensation for their services, and empowers them to contribute meaningfully to the healthcare ecosystem. Only through such comprehensive reforms can the dignity, value, and crucial role of nurses be restored in Nigeria's healthcare landscape.

Chapter Six

A CRY FOR RECOGNITION

Recognizing and celebrating the exceptional contributions of Nigerian nurses will play pivotal in restoring the dignity and value of the nursing profession. Establishing robust structures and mechanisms for acknowledging the efforts and achievements of exceptional nurses is essential to uplift their morale and inspire a sense of pride in their work. Not all nurses can be recognized, that is just the fundamental truth. Not all actors are recognized, not all musicians are recognized, but the ones that get the required recognition inspires those who don't get recognition. That is the ultimate goal.

Nurses are the backbone of the healthcare system. Their dedication, expertise, and unwavering commitment to patient care often go unnoticed or underappreciated. However, creating avenues for recognition can transform the narrative, fostering a culture that appreciates and values the critical role nurses play in healthcare delivery. One way to achieve this, is through the establishment of awards, honors, or merit-based recognition programs specifically designed to celebrate the accomplishments of nurses. Recognizing excellence in various specialties, innovative practices, leadership, research, and community service within nursing can elevate the profile of the profession and motivate nurses to strive for excellence.

Moreover, initiatives such as nurse-of-the-year awards, exemplary service recognitions, or spotlighting successful projects undertaken by nurses can provide a platform to showcase their contributions. These recognitions not only honour individual achievements but also serve as inspiration for others, fostering a culture of continuous improvement and excellence within the nursing community. In addition to awards, creating platforms for sharing success stories, highlighting the impact of nurses' efforts, and amplifying their voices in healthcare discourse can be immensely empowering. Events, conferences, or forums dedicated to nursing achievements can provide visibility and acknowledgment for the remarkable work done by nurses across diverse settings. Also, investing in professional development opportunities, such as scholarships, grants, or fellowships, for nurses who demonstrate exceptional promise or innovation can encourage a culture of ongoing learning and advancement within the profession.

Statistics and examples from countries with successful recognition programs for nurses can serve as models to emulate. For instance, countries like the United States, Canada, or Australia have established prestigious nursing awards that honor outstanding contributions, innovative practices, and leadership within the nursing field. These programs not only boost morale but also attract talented individuals to the profession and promote a positive image of nursing in society. Unity and cohesion among nurses are crucial for the advancement and recognition of the profession. Establishing a unified and cohesive body within nursing not only fosters solidarity but also strengthens the collective voice of nurses, advocating for their rights, professional development, and the enhancement of healthcare services.

Emphasizing professionalism and continuous improvement beyond certificates is crucial. It's about instilling a culture of lifelong learning, ethical conduct, and commitment to excellence. Respecting every licensed nurse, regardless of their educational background or specialization, is the key to a culture of inclusivity and mutual respect within the nursing fraternity. Moreover, when nurses stand united under a single, cohesive entity, they have a stronger voice to address systemic challenges, advocate for policy changes that benefit both nurses and patients, and contribute to shaping the future of healthcare.

Then again, the concept of a unified nursing body transcends individual certificates or qualifications; it's about promoting professionalism, collaboration, and continuous improvement in service delivery. When nurses come together under a single, unified organization or body, they amplify their collective influence and facilitate concerted efforts towards common goals. A unified nursing body can advocate for the rights and welfare of nurses, ensuring fair compensation, improved working conditions, and avenues for career advancement. Moreso speaking with a unified voice, nurses can effectively address issues affecting the profession, such as regulatory reforms, standardization of practices, and policies that impact patient care. Such unified bodies can provide a platform for continuous professional development, offering educational resources, training opportunities, and mentorship programs.

These initiatives are pivotal in promoting a culture of lifelong learning among nurses, enhancing their skills, and keeping them abreast of advancements in healthcare practices.

Countries with strong nursing associations or unions serve as examples of the positive impact of unified bodies within the nursing profession. For instance, nursing associations in various countries like the American Nurses Association (ANA) in the United States, the Royal College of Nursing (RCN) in the United Kingdom, or the Canadian Nurses Association (CNA) have been instrumental in advocating for nurses' rights, shaping healthcare policies, and promoting professional growth.

Respecting every licensed nurse and recognizing their contributions to healthcare is fundamental. Regardless of their level of experience or specialization, every licensed nurse deserves respect, acknowledgment, and support in their professional journey. Valuing each nurse's expertise and unique contributions contributes to a positive work environment, fostering a culture of mutual respect and collaboration.

Chapter Seven

POLICY PARALYSIS: NAVIGATING BUREAUCRATIC BARRIERS

P olicy paralysis within Nigeria's healthcare sector serves as a catalyst for the myriad challenges faced by nurses and the broader healthcare system. This stagnation in policy formulation, implementation, and adaptation hampers progress and exacerbates the existing loopholes, undermining the potential for meaningful reforms and improvements. The health sector in Nigeria grapples with deep-rooted policy paralysis characterized by a lack of coherent, adaptive, and effectively implemented policies. The failure to enact and enforce robust policies results in systemic inadequacies, including insufficient budgetary allocations, ineffective resource distribution, and a dearth of sustainable strategies to address healthcare challenges.

For instance, the persistent failure to meet the commitment of allocating 15% of the national budget to healthcare, as pledged by the African Union in 2001, exemplifies this policy paralysis. Despite the potential transformative impact of such financial commitment, Nigeria consistently falls short, allocating a fraction of the recommended budget to healthcare, leading to inadequate infrastructure, limited access to essential medicines, and a lack of adequate resources for healthcare professionals.

Navigating bureaucratic barriers further compounds the challenges. The corridors of power in Nigeria are often marred by bureaucratic red tape, inefficiencies, and systemic complexities that impede the timely implementation of healthcare policies. This bureaucratic maze creates bottlenecks, delaying decision-making processes, hindering effective resource allocation, and stalling initiatives aimed at improving healthcare delivery. Corruption, vested interests, and a lack of political will within bureaucratic structures hinder the swift implementation of reforms critical for transforming the healthcare sector. The intricate web of bureaucratic hurdles often sidelines urgent healthcare needs, perpetuating the status quo of inadequate infrastructure, underfunded facilities, and demotivated healthcare professionals.

To illustrate, the slow implementation of policies that prioritize healthcare infrastructure development, equitable resource allocation, and adequate remuneration for healthcare workers showcases the bureaucratic challenges that impede progress. Despite the pressing need for such reforms, bureaucratic complexities and vested interests derail or delay these crucial initiatives, perpetuating the cycle of systemic inadequacies.

Addressing policy paralysis and navigating bureaucratic barriers in Nigeria's healthcare sector requires multifaceted solutions. There is an urgent need for political commitment to enact and enforce policies that prioritize healthcare, allocating adequate resources, and ensuring effective implementation. Additionally, streamlining bureaucratic processes, enhancing transparency, and promoting accountability within governmental structures are imperative to facilitate efficient decision-making and expedite reforms. Navigating bureaucratic barriers within Nigeria's corridors of power further exacerbates these challenges.

Bureaucratic hurdles, red tape, and administrative complexities create obstacles that impede swift decision-making and effective policy implementation within the healthcare sector:

1. **Complex Administrative Procedures:** Cumbersome bureaucratic procedures hinder the efficient functioning of healthcare institutions. Obtaining approvals, accessing resources, or initiating reforms often involve confusing processes that delay progress.

2. **Corruption and Mismanagement:** The prevalence of corruption and mismanagement within bureaucratic structures siphons resources away from essential healthcare needs. Funds intended for healthcare improvements might be misappropriated, leading to a lack of necessary infrastructure, equipment, or training for nurses.

3. **Lack of Coordination and Collaboration:** Fragmented governance structures and a lack of coordination among different levels of government and relevant stakeholders result in disjointed efforts. This disorganization often leads to duplication of efforts, inefficiencies, and a failure to address critical healthcare challenges comprehensively.

4. **Political Interference:** The healthcare sector sometimes falls victim to political interests, leading to policy decisions driven more by political agendas rather than healthcare needs. This interference can hinder the implementation of evidence-based policies and reforms beneficial to the nursing profession.

In essence, policy paralysis and bureaucratic barriers hinder the effective functioning of Nigeria's healthcare system, impeding progress in addressing the myriad challenges faced by nurses. Addressing these issues demands a concerted effort to streamline policies, enhance regulatory frameworks, combat corruption, and foster collaboration among stakeholders to create a conducive environment for the nursing profession to thrive and contribute meaningfully to healthcare delivery. Models from other countries that have successfully overcome similar bureaucratic barriers through streamlined processes, anti-corruption measures, and strategic policy reforms can serve as guiding examples. Reforming the bureaucratic system to prioritize the healthcare sector's needs is pivotal to fostering an environment conducive to transformative policy changes that can uplift the nursing profession and improve healthcare outcomes for all Nigerians.

Chapter Eight

THE RIPPLE EFFECT: IMPACT ON PATIENT CARE

The repercussions of the challenges faced by nurses in Nigeria trickle down to affect patients profoundly. The strain, frustration, and limitations experienced by nurses due to systemic issues directly impact patient care, leading to suboptimal outcomes and a compromised healthcare experience.

1. **Quality of Care:** The systemic issues and constraints faced by nurses often result in a diminished quality of care for patients. When nurses are overworked, underappreciated, or lacking necessary resources and support, their ability to provide optimal care is compromised. Patients might experience longer wait times, rushed consultations, or incomplete attention to their needs, which affects their overall satisfaction with the healthcare system.

2. **Communication and Attitude:** The negative environment within healthcare settings can manifest in the attitudes and communication styles of nurses. While the majority of nurses strive to provide compassionate care, the strain of their working conditions might inadvertently lead to perceived rudeness or lack of

empathy. Patients, unfortunately, might interpret this as a reflection of the nursing profession as a whole. The stress and burnout experienced by nurses can affect the quality of their interactions, leaving patients feeling neglected or disregarded.

3. **Impact on Mental Health:** The distress and depression experienced by nurses due to their challenges seep into their interactions with patients. Nurses dealing with their own stress might find it difficult to maintain a positive demeanor, impacting the emotional support they provide to patients. This, in turn, affects the mental well-being of patients who require not just physical care but also emotional reassurance.

4. **Longer Wait Times and Delayed Care:** Insufficient staffing, administrative hurdles,

and bureaucratic inefficiencies can lead to longer wait times for patients seeking healthcare services. Delayed care due to these systemic issues can worsen health conditions, compromise timely interventions, and contribute to negative health outcomes.

5. **Continuity of Care:** Inconsistent staffing levels, high turnover rates, and limited resources can disrupt the continuity of care for patients. When nurses are unable to practice their specialties or are constantly overwhelmed, patients might not receive consistent and coordinated care, leading to fragmented treatment and potential gaps in their healthcare journey.

6. **Inadequate Facilities and Resources:** Patients may face challenges accessing necessary facilities, medications, or specialized

care due to systemic deficiencies in the healthcare infrastructure. Lack of essential medical supplies, outdated equipment, or insufficient beds in hospitals can directly impact patient treatment and recovery.

7. **Psychological Impact:** The overall environment within healthcare settings, influenced by systemic challenges and stressed healthcare workers, can have a significant psychological impact on patients. Patients may feel anxious, disheartened, or distressed due to the perceived inadequacies in care delivery and the overall atmosphere in healthcare facilities.

Statistics and reports from patient satisfaction surveys or healthcare quality assessments can further highlight the correlation between systemic nursing challenges and patient experiences. Such data often reflect patient dissatisfaction with healthcare services, increased incidences of medical errors, longer hospital stays, and overall concerns about the quality of care provided. In essence, the challenges faced by nurses directly have a lasting effect on the patient experience. Addressing the systemic issues within the nursing profession is crucial not only for the well-being of nurses themselves but also for improving patient outcomes, enhancing the quality of care delivered, and fostering a more compassionate and patient-centered healthcare system.

While acknowledging that there might be a few individuals whose behaviour doesn't align with the nursing profession's ethics, it's crucial to recognize that the larger systemic issues create an environment that makes it challenging for nurses to consistently deliver the level of care they aspire to provide.

Chapter Nine

VOICES FROM THE FRONTLINE

The call for change within the nursing profession in Nigeria requires collective action from every nurse, regardless of their socioeconomic status or hierarchical position within the healthcare system. Nurses possess a unique vantage point and firsthand experience of the challenges that plague the healthcare system. Embracing this role as advocates for change can spark transformative initiatives and contribute to much-needed reforms. Consider the following:

1. **Utilizing Collective Strength:** Nurses, by banding together, can leverage their collective strength to advocate for systemic changes. Initiating or joining professional associations, nursing forums, or advocacy groups allows nurses to amplify their voices and work collaboratively towards addressing key issues. These organizations provide platforms for collaboration, knowledge sharing, and collective advocacy for policy changes that benefit the nursing workforce and patient care. When unified, nurses become a formidable force for advocating policy reforms, better working conditions, and improved patient care standards.

1. I have found a way to champion this course. I did this by setting up the COA Connect, an organization that is set on empowering Nigerian nurses, redefining the nursing profession through education and active nursing-centric initiatives, and celebrating nurses achievements.

2. **Advocacy and Awareness:** Nurses can leverage their collective voice and advocacy skills to raise awareness about systemic issues affecting the profession. Engaging in discussions, seminars, or public forums, and utilizing social media platforms can amplify their voices and draw attention to critical issues such as inadequate staffing, lack of resources, or substandard working conditions.

3. **Being Agents of Change:** Nurses don't need positions of power to drive change; they can

create impactful transformations through their actions in everyday practice. Implementing small-scale initiatives within their spheres of influence can create ripples of change. For instance, promoting patient education, fostering a culture of empathy and respect, or advocating for better infection control measures within their units.

4. **Engaging in Advocacy and Education:** Nurses can engage in community outreach programs, health education campaigns, or public awareness initiatives to highlight healthcare issues. By educating the public, policymakers, and fellow healthcare professionals about the challenges faced and the potential solutions, nurses can garner support for much-needed reforms.

5. **Quality Improvement Initiatives:** Nurses, irrespective of their roles, can actively participate in quality improvement initiatives within their healthcare settings. They can contribute ideas, suggest process improvements, and actively engage in implementing changes aimed at enhancing patient care, safety, and overall healthcare delivery.

6. **Using Social Media and Technology:** Leveraging the power of social media platforms and digital tools can amplify nurses' voices. Sharing personal experiences, raising awareness about systemic issues, and advocating for change through online platforms can reach a wider audience and garner public support for reforms.

7. **Community Engagement:** Engaging with local communities and patients allows nurses

to understand their needs better. By being involved in community health programs, health education initiatives, or volunteering activities, nurses can contribute to improving health outcomes beyond the hospital setting.

5. **Educational Initiatives:** Nurses can take the initiative to educate themselves and others on best practices, evidence-based care, and professional development opportunities. This continuous learning and knowledge-sharing culture can significantly impact the quality of care provided.

Examples abound for nurses across the globe initiating impactful changes:

- In the United States, grassroots movements led by nurses have influenced policy changes, such as improved nurse-patient ratios and better workplace safety standards.

- In India, nurses have championed initiatives to improve sanitation practices and infection control in healthcare settings, significantly reducing hospital-acquired infections.

While statistical data may not quantify the direct impact of individual nurses' efforts in effecting change, anecdotal evidence and success stories exist where nurses, through their determination and collective action, have influenced positive transformations in healthcare settings. Instances of successful advocacy campaigns, quality improvement projects leading to enhanced patient care, or community health initiatives resulting in improved health outcomes can be found through testimonials and case studies.

Ultimately, the collective actions of individual nurses, when united by a common goal of advancing the nursing profession and improving patient care, can create a ripple effect that drives meaningful change within the healthcare system. Every nurse has the potential to be an agent of change by utilizing their skills, knowledge, and passion for the betterment of healthcare delivery.

Chapter Ten

A PRESCRIPTION FOR CHANGE

T he cries for change within the nursing profession echo as a collective plea for a reformed system, one that liberates rather than constrains, fosters growth instead of stagnation, and fundamentally enhances the quality of healthcare for all. It's a resounding demand to shatter the shackles that confine nursing autonomy and a fervent call to acknowledge and empower nurses for their indispensable role. Consider the following:

1. Empowerment through Autonomy

Studies have shown that healthcare systems that grant nurses greater autonomy witness a significant surge in patient outcomes. Research by renowned institutions like the World Health Organization (WHO) and the American Nurses Association (ANA) underscores that increased nursing autonomy directly correlates with reduced mortality rates, lowered infection rates, and improved patient satisfaction scores. According to the World Health Organization (WHO), nurses form the largest segment of the global healthcare workforce, accounting for nearly 59% of health professionals. Furthermore, studies reveal that an increase in the nurse-to-patient ratio correlates with reduced mortality rates, shorter hospital stays, and improved patient outcomes. In essence, empowering nurses translates directly to enhancing the quality and efficiency of healthcare services.

2. Global Success Stories

Across various high-performing healthcare systems, such as those in Scandinavian countries and certain regions of Canada, where nurses are granted substantial autonomy in decision-making, statistics exhibit an unparalleled level of healthcare excellence. For instance, in Norway, where nurses have a high degree of autonomy, they have prescriptive authority and independent practice, healthcare indices are consistently ranked among the top worldwide, showcasing the transformative potential of nursing empowerment. Patient satisfaction rates soar, and the healthcare system witnesses greater efficiency and cost-effectiveness. Similarly, in Switzerland, the implementation of advanced nursing roles and expanded scopes of practice has elevated the standard of care.

3. Financial Advantages

Beyond enhanced patient outcomes, granting nurses autonomy has also demonstrated economic benefits. Reports from healthcare economies like Australia and the Netherlands reveal that empowering nurses with greater decision-making authority will not only elevate care standards but also generate cost-efficiency through reduced hospital readmissions and shorter patient stays.

4. Retention and Job Satisfaction

The correlation between nursing autonomy and job satisfaction cannot be overstated. Data from Gallup Polls and employee satisfaction surveys indicate that nurses working in environments that value their autonomy exhibit higher job fulfillment, leading to reduced turnover rates and a more sustainable healthcare workforce.

In light of these robust findings, it's evident that the paradigm shift toward granting nurses the autonomy they deserve isn't just a moral imperative but an evidence-based necessity. When nurses are empowered to exercise their expertise, ingenuity, and compassion, the very essence of superior healthcare unfolds.

The collective outcry from nurses resonates as a poignant call for a transformative shift in the healthcare landscape. It echoes a resounding demand for a system that not only acknowledges the tireless efforts of nurses but also empowers them to wield their expertise without shackles. The time has come to dismantle the barriers that hinder nursing autonomy and obstruct the delivery of quality care. Granting autonomy to nurses isn't just a matter of empowerment; it's a testament to recognizing their invaluable contributions. Research published in reputable medical journals demonstrates a clear correlation between nursing autonomy and patient safety. Studies from the Journal of Nursing Administration and the Institute of Medicine reveal that empowering nurses with autonomy in decision-making results in fewer medical errors, reduced hospital-acquired infections, and enhanced overall patient safety.

The call for change is not merely a plea; it's a strategic imperative for healthcare systems worldwide. It's about acknowledging the wealth of knowledge, skills, and compassion that nurses bring to the table and creating an environment where these attributes can flourish. Autonomy is the cornerstone upon which nurses can exercise their expertise, innovate care delivery, and steer the healthcare trajectory towards excellence.

Chapter Eleven

RAISING THE FLAG: ADVOCACY AND ACTIVISM

The flag for nursing advocacy and activism is more than a call for autonomy; it's a rallying cry for the right to bring about transformative change in patient care. Nurses aren't just seeking freedom; they're yearning for the opportunity to leverage their expertise, intuition, and skillset to make pivotal decisions that can be life-altering for patients. Their impassioned plea resonates as a plea for liberation within the healthcare system—a system that should champion their ability to innovate, personalize care, and foster healing beyond mere treatment.

Consider the significance of nurse-led initiatives and advocacy efforts globally. The "Nightingale Model of Care" in the United Kingdom, founded on the principles of whole care, empathy, and patient-centeredness, exemplifies the impact of nurse-driven approaches. The model not only emphasizes patient advocacy but also underscores the importance of empowering nurses to make clinical decisions in alignment with their expertise. As a result, it has yielded improved patient satisfaction, reduced readmission rates, and enhanced overall healthcare quality.

In Canada, nurses rallied for legislative changes that granted them expanded roles in primary care and allowed nurse practitioners to independently diagnose and prescribe medications. The result? Enhanced access to healthcare services, improved patient outcomes, and a more robust, patient-centered healthcare system. Also, in Australia, nursing advocacy movements have led to policy reforms that recognize nurses' pivotal role in healthcare decision-making. Their concerted efforts have resulted in progressive shifts towards a healthcare model that values and empowers nurses' professional judgment. These changes have not only elevated the status of nursing but have also elevated the quality of care delivered to patients across the nation. Nurse practitioners are granted prescriptive authority and independent practice, by illustrating the profound impact of trusting nurses with greater responsibility. Studies from the Australian Journal of Advanced Nursing reveal that enhanced autonomy leads to increased patient satisfaction, better access to care, and improved health outcomes.

Nursing advocacy and activism are pivotal in reshaping the healthcare narrative. Examples abound where nurses, through tireless advocacy, have influenced policy changes, introduced innovative care models, and spearheaded transformative reforms. From advocating for improved nurse-to-patient ratios to pushing for legislative changes to recognize advanced nursing roles, their concerted efforts have sparked tangible improvements in healthcare delivery.

Nursing advocacy is not confined to legislative battles alone; it thrives in the daily interactions between nurses and their patients. It's the nurse who advocates tirelessly for a patient's well-being, they ensure that their unique needs are met beyond medical treatment. It's the nurse who speaks up for patient rights, ensures informed consent, and champions a compassionate approach to care. The heart of nursing advocacy beats louder with every instance where nurses tailor care to suit individual patients, recognizing their cultural nuances, beliefs, and preferences. It's about transcending the cookie-cutter approach and embracing a patient-centric model that acknowledges the humanity within healthcare.

This call for advocacy and activism isn't just about nurses; it's about patients. It's about a healthcare system that truly values the expertise and dedication of those on the frontlines. Nurses yearn for a healthcare ethos that honours their professional judgment, fosters trust, and unleashes their potential to not just treat ailments but to heal the whole person.

Nurses cry for trust, recognition, and autonomy is not a mere request in Nigeria—it's a clarion call for a healthcare system that liberates nurses from constraints and empowers them to exercise their professional judgment. It's about creating an environment where nurses are not just seen as caregivers but as instrumental leaders in driving healthcare excellence. It's a profound plea for a system that not only acknowledges their expertise but also celebrates their unwavering commitment to healing, compassion, and patient-centric care. Ultimately, nurse-led advocacy and activism serve as catalysts for transformative change, fostering a healthcare landscape that respects, values, and harnesses the unparalleled potential of nurses in delivering quality, and patient-centered care.

Chapter Twelve

A FUTURE FOR NIGERIAN NURSES

L ooking ahead, the future for Nigerian nurses brims with the promise of transformation and resurgence. Having unearthed the deep-rooted challenges plaguing the nursing profession, outlined viable solutions, and illuminated a path forward, the horizon is ripe for change. Nigerian nurses stand poised at the threshold of a new era, one that champions their expertise, empowers their voices, and nurtures their growth.

It's a future where the scars of policy paralysis are healed by proactive governance and strategic reforms. As seen in countries like the United Kingdom and Sweden, where investment in nursing education and improved working conditions has resulted in heightened job satisfaction and superior patient outcomes, Nigeria too can chart a similar course.

For this future to materialize, a concerted effort is imperative. The government must translate pledges into action by allocating a substantial budget to healthcare, ensuring the equitable distribution of resources, and fostering a supportive environment for nursing practice. It's about establishing mechanisms that recognize and reward nurses for their dedication, commitment, and continuous learning.

Nurses themselves are integral to shaping this future. Through active involvement in professional associations, continuous education, and embracing leadership roles, they can drive the narrative of change within their ranks. Embracing innovation, advocating for nursing autonomy, and fostering a culture of collaboration and mentorship will be pivotal in shaping a resilient and empowered nursing workforce. The blueprint for this future extends beyond the confines of hospitals and clinics. It encompasses community engagement, tapping into traditional medicine, and leveraging technology to bridge healthcare gaps. Initiatives like integrating therapeutic gardens in healthcare facilities, investing in local drug production, and adopting patient-centered care models are crucial components that can revolutionize healthcare delivery in Nigeria.

Statistics and success stories from progressive healthcare systems worldwide serve as beacons of hope. When the system values its nurses, it reaps the dividends in enhanced patient outcomes, reduced healthcare costs, and an overall upliftment of societal well-being. The path ahead is illuminated by the collective resolve to address challenges, embrace innovation, and advocate for a healthcare system that places nurses at its core. It's not just a future for Nigerian nurses; it's a future where healthcare is defined by compassion, expertise, and a relentless commitment to human dignity. As these seeds of transformation take root, the promise of a brighter tomorrow for Nigerian nurses stands ready to blossom into a reality.

ACKNOWLEDGEMENTS

First of all, my profound gratitude goes to God Almighty for the grace He has bestowed upon me and all that concerns me. I deeply appreciate my dear husband, Chief, Adeyeri Stephen Kunle, for being my support system during the writing of this book. Thanks to my parents, Mr. and Mrs. Stephen Okafor, for bringing up an open-minded, brilliant daughter, and for funding my chosen discipline: nursing. Thank you, daddy and mummy, for teaching me the act of service and impacting the lives of others. A big thank you to my twin sister Engr Winifred Okafor for always supporting every of my ideas and for encouraging me when I picked up my pen to write this book.

REFERENCES

Chapter 1

- Askia-Williams laments plight of Nigerian nurses. (2016, July 2nd). Nigerian Tribune. https://tribuneonlineng.com/regina-askia-williams-laments-plight-nigerian-nurses/ Retrieved Nov. 29th, 2023.

- Kene, O. (2022, May 20th) The Plight And Flight Of Nigerian Health Workers Opinion Nigeria. https://www.opinionnigeria.com/the-plight-and-flight-of-nigerian-health-workers-by-kene-obiezu/, Retrieved 30th Nov., 2023.

- Vote 15% of budget to health, doctors urge Tinubu (2023, Nov., 6th) Punch. https://punchng.com/vote-15-of-budget-to-health-doctors-urge-tinubu/#:~:text=The%20Abuja%20Declaration%20commitment%20requires,neglected%20in%20the%20supplementary%20budget, Retrieved 30th Nov., 2023.

Chapter 2

- Better Health Channel. (2015, Oct. 18th) Visitors in Hospital Better Health Channel. https://www.betterhealth.vic.gov.au/health/servicesandsupport/visitors-in-hospital, Retrieved 29th Nov., 2023.

Chapter 3

- 2023 Budget: Health gets highest allocation ever but fails to meet AU commitment (2022, Oct. 12th). Premium Times. https://www.premiumtimesng.com/news/headlines/559213-2023-budget-health-gets-highest-allocation-ever-but-fails-to-meet-au-commitment.html?tztc=1, Retrieved 30th Nov., 2023.

- Here's Why GSK is Leaving Nigeria After 51 Years (2023, Aug. 8th). TheCable. https://www.thecable.ng/explainer-heres-why-gsk-is-leaving-nigeria-after-51-years, Retrieved 30th Nov., 2023.

Chapter 4

- Nursing and Midwifery Council of Nigeria (2023, Aug. 21st) Wikipedia. https://en.wikipedia.org/wiki/Nursing_and_Midwifery_Council_of_Nigeria#:~:text=Originally%20founded%20in%201949%20as,89%2C%201979, Retrieved 1st Dec., 2023.

- Brandy G. NurseJournal Staff (2023, Aug., 24th) Types of Nursing Degrees and Levels NurseJournal. https://nursejournal.org/degrees/types-of-nursing-degrees/, Retrieved 1st Dec., 2023.

Chapter 7

- Nigeria - Country Commercial Guide. (2023, June 6th) https://www.trade.gov/country-commercial-guides/nigeria-healthcare#:~:text=The%20Nigerian%20healthcare%20industry%20is,budget%20to%20health%20in%202021%2C, International Trade Administration. Retrieved 2nd Dec., 2023.

Chapter 9

- Ester C., Charles S. (2004, November 3rd). Nurses and Labor Activism in the United States: The Role of Class, Gender, and Ideology Jstor. https://www.jstor.org/stable/29768259, Retrieved 1st Dec., 2023.

- Flaubert JL, Le Menestrel S, Williams DR. (2021, May 11th) The Future of Nursing 2020-2030: Charting a Path to Achieve Health Equity National Library of Medicine. https://www.ncbi.nlm.nih.gov/books/NBK573918/, Retrieved 30th Nov., 2023.

Chapter 10

- Nursing and Midwifery. (2023) https://www.who.int/health-topics/nursing#tab=tab_1, World Health Organization. Retrieved 2nd Dec., 2023.

- Nurses Retain Top Ethics Rating in U.S., but Below 2020 High (2023 10th Jan.) https://news.gallup.com/poll/467804/nurses-retain-top-ethics-rating-below-2020-high.aspx, Gallup. Retrieved 2nd Dec., 2023.

Chapter 11

- Florence Nightingale: Environmental Theory (2023 2nd July) https://nurseslabs.com/florence-nightingales-environmental-theory/, Nurselabs. Retrieved 2nd Dec., 2023.

Chapter 5, 6, 8, 12

- Nil